RENAL DIET COOKBOOK

40+ Recipes: Seafood and Smoothies

How to Take Control of Your Kidney Disease and Avoid Dialysis.

Irene Simmons

Table of Contents

Introduction

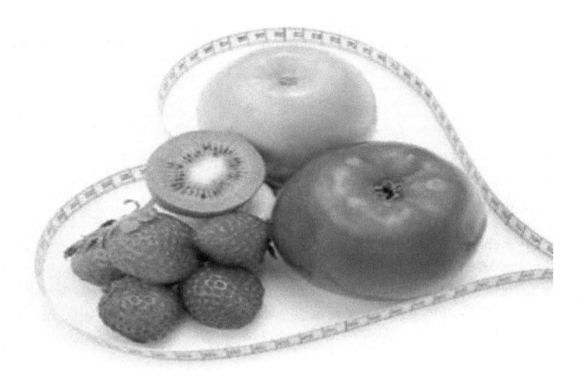

Human health hangs in a complete balance when all of its interconnected bodily mechanisms function properly in perfect sync. Without its major organs working normally, the body soon suffers indelible damage. Kidney malfunction is one such example, and it is not just the entire water balance that is disturbed by the kidney disease, but a number of other diseases also emerge due to this problem. Kidney diseases are progressive in nature, meaning that if left unchecked and uncontrolled, they can ultimately lead to permanent kidney damage. That is why it is essential to control and manage the disease and put a halt to its progress, which can be done through medicinal and natural means. While medicines can guarantee only thirty percent of the cure, a change of lifestyle and diet can prove to be miraculous with seventy percent of guaranteed results. A kidney-friendly diet and lifestyle not only saves the kidneys from excess minerals but they also aid medicines to work actively. Treatment without a good diet, hence, proves to be useless. In this renal diet cookbook, we shall bring out the basic facts about kidney diseases, their symptoms, causes, and diagnosis. This preliminary introduction can help the readers understand the problem clearly; then, we shall discuss the role of renal diet and kidney-friendly lifestyle in curbing the diseases. And it's not just that. The book also contains a range of delicious renal diet recipes that will guarantee luscious flavors and good health.

Despite their tiny size, the kidneys perform a number of functions, which are vital for the body to be able to function healthily.

These include:

- Filtering excess fluids and waste from the blood
- Creating the enzyme known as renin, which regulates blood pressure,
- Ensuring bone marrow creates red blood cells,
- Controlling calcium and phosphorus levels through absorption and excretion.

Unfortunately, when kidney disease reaches a chronic stage, these functions start to stop working. However, with the right treatment and lifestyle, it is possible to manage symptoms and continue living well. This is even more applicable in the earlier stages of the disease. Tactlessly, 10% of all adults over the age of 20 will experience some form of kidney disease in their lifetime. There are a variety of different treatments for kidney disease, which depend on the cause of the disease.

Kidney (or renal) diseases are affecting around 14% of the adult population, according to international stats. In the US, approx. 661.000 Americans suffer from kidney dysfunction. Out of these patients, 468.000 proceed to dialysis treatment, and the rest have one active kidney transplant.

The high quantities of diabetes and heart illness are additionally related to kidney dysfunction, and sometimes one condition, for example, diabetes, may prompt the other.

With such a significant number of high rates, possibly the best course of treatment is the contravention of dialysis, which makes people depend upon clinical and crisis facility meds on any occasion multiple times every week. In this manner, if your kidney has just given a few indications of brokenness, you can forestall dialysis through an eating routine, something that we will talk about in this book.

What to Know About the Kidney Disease

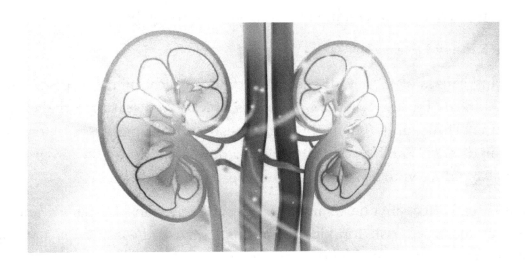

Kidney disease is becoming more prevalent in the United States, and so we need to learn as much about it as we can. The more we educate ourselves, the more we can do to take care of this important bodily system. If you've been diagnosed with chronic kidney disease (CKD), education can empower you to most effectively and purposefully manage the disease. Once you have a full understanding of what chronic kidney disease is, you can begin to take charge of your evolving health needs. Making healthy changes early in the stages of kidney disease will help determine how well you will manage your kidney health. I am here to guide you, every step of the way. Like any new process, it may seem intimidating at first. But this chapter provides the foundation for learning, and will help you understand kidney disease as you begin your journey to healthier kidneys.

What Do the Kidneys Do?

Our kidneys are small, but they do powerful things to keep our body in balance. They are bean-shaped, about the size of a fist, and are located in the middle of the back, on the left and right sides of the spine, just below the rib cage. When everything is working properly, the kidneys do many important jobs such as:

- Filter waste materials from the blood

- Remove extra fluid, or water, from the body
- Release hormones that help manage blood pressure
- Stimulate bone marrow to make red blood cells
- Make an active form of vitamin D that promotes strong, healthy bones

What Causes Kidney Disease?

There are many causes of kidney disease, including physical injury or disorders that can damage the kidneys, but the two leading causes of kidney disease are diabetes and high blood pressure. These underlying conditions also put people at risk for developing cardiovascular disease. Early treatment may not only slow down the progression of the disease, but also reduce your risk of developing heart disease or stroke.

Kidney disease can affect anyone, at any age. African Americans, Hispanics, and American Indians are at increased risk for kidney failure, because these groups have a greater prevalence of diabetes and high blood pressure.

When we digest protein, our bodies create waste products. As blood flows through the capillaries, the waste products are filtered through the urine. Substances such as protein and red blood cells are too big to pass through the capillaries and so stay in the blood. All the extra work takes a toll on the kidneys. When kidney disease is detected in the early stages, several treatments may prevent the worsening of the disease. If kidney disease is detected in the later stages, high amounts of protein in your urine, called macro albuminuria, can lead to end-stage renal disease.

The second leading cause of kidney disease is high blood pressure, also known as hypertension. One in three Americans is at risk for kidney disease because of hypertension. Although there is no cure for hypertension, certain medications, a low-sodium diet, and physical activity can lower blood pressure.

The kidneys help manage blood pressure, but when blood pressure is high, the heart has to work overtime at pumping blood. When the force of blood flow is high, blood vessels start to stretch so the blood can flow more easily. The stretching and scarring weakens the blood vessels throughout the entire body, including the kidneys. And when the kidneys' blood vessels are injured, they may not remove the waste and extra fluid from the body, creating a dangerous cycle, because the extra fluid in the blood vessels can increase blood pressure even more.

With diabetes, excess blood sugar remains in the bloodstream. The high blood sugar levels can damage the blood vessels in the kidneys and elsewhere in the body. And since high blood pressure is a complication from diabetes, the extra pressure can weaken the walls of the blood vessels, which can lead to a heart attack or stroke.

Other conditions, such as drug abuse and certain autoimmune diseases, can also cause injury to the kidneys. In fact, every drug we put into our body has to pass through the kidneys for filtration.

An autoimmune disease is one in which the immune system, designed to protect the body from illness, sees the body as an invader and attacks its own systems, including the kidneys. Some forms of lupus, for example, attack the kidneys. Another autoimmune disease that can lead to kidney failure is Good pasture syndrome, a group of conditions that affect the kidneys and the lungs. The damage to the kidneys from autoimmune diseases can lead to chronic kidney disease and kidney failure.

Treatment Plans for Chronic Kidney Disease (Cod)

The best way to manage CKD is to be an active participant in your treatment program, regardless of your stage of renal disease. Proper treatment involves a combination of working with a healthcare team, adhering to a renal diet, and making healthy lifestyle decisions. These can all have a profoundly positive effect on your kidney disease—especially watching how you eat.

Working with your healthcare team. When you have kidney disease, working in partnership with your healthcare team can be extremely important in your treatment program as well as being personally empowering. Regularly meeting with your physician or healthcare team can arm you with resources and information that help you make informed decisions regarding your treatment needs, and provide you with a much needed opportunity to vent, share information, get advice, and receive support in effectively managing this illness.

Adhering to a renal diet. The heart of this book is the renal diet. Sticking to this diet can make a huge difference in your health and vitality. Like any change, following the diet may not be easy at first. Important changes to your diet, particularly early on, can possibly prevent the need for dialysis. These changes include limiting salt, eating a low-protein diet, reducing fat intake, and getting enough calories if you need to lose weight. Be honest with yourself first and foremost—learn what you need, and consider your personal goals and obstacles. Start by making small changes. It is okay to have some slip-ups—we all do. With guidance and support, these small changes will become habits of your promising new lifestyle. In no time, you will begin taking control of your diet and health.

Making healthy lifestyle decisions. Lifestyle choices play a crucial part in our health, especially when it comes to helping regulate kidney disease. Lifestyle choices such as allotting time for physical activity, getting enough sleep, managing weight, reducing stress, and limiting smoking and alcohol will help you take control of your overall health, making it easier to manage your kidney disease. Follow this simple formula: Keep toxins out of your body as much as you can, and build up your immune system with a good balance of exercise, relaxation, and sleep.

What to do to Slow down Kidney Disease

A kidney disease diagnosis can seem devastating at first. The news may come as a shock for some people, who may not have experienced any symptoms. It's important to remember that you can control your progress and improvement through diet and lifestyle changes, even when a prognosis is serious. Taking steps to improve your health can make a significant effort to slow the progression of kidney disease and improve your quality of life.

Focus on Weight Loss

Losing weight is one of the most common reasons for going on a diet. It's also one of the best ways to treat kidney disease and prevent further damage. Carrying excess weight contributes to high toxicity levels in the body, by storing toxins instead of releasing them through the kidneys. Eating foods high in trans fats, sugar, and excess sodium contribute to obesity, which affects close to one third of North Americans and continues to rise in many other countries, where fast foods are becoming easier to access and less expensive. Losing weight is a difficult cycle for many, who often diet temporarily only to return to unhealthy habits after reaching a milestone, which results in gaining the weight back, thus causing an unhealthy "yo-yo" diet effect.

There are some basic and easy changes you can make to shed those first pounds, which will begin to take the pressure off the kidneys and help you onto the path of regular weight loss:

Drink plenty of water. If you can't drink eight glasses a day, try adding unsweetened natural sparkling water or herbal teas to increase your water intake.

Reduce the amount of sugar and carbohydrates you consume. This doesn't require adapting to a ketogenic or low-carb diet – you'll notice a major change after ditching soda and reducing the bread and pasta by half.

Take your time to eat and avoid rushing. If you need to eat in a hurry, grab a piece of fruit or a small portion of macadamia nuts. Avoid sugary and salty foods as much as possible. Choose fresh fruits over potato chips and chocolate bars.

Create a short list of kidney-friendly foods that you enjoy and use this as your reference or guide when grocery shopping. This will help you stock up on snacks, ingredients, and foods for your kitchen that work well within your renal diet plan, at the same time reducing your chances of succumbing to the temptation of eating a bag of salted pretzels or chocolate.

Once you make take a few steps towards changing the way you eat, it will get easier. Making small changes at first is the key to success and to progressing with a new way of eating and living. If you are already in the habit of consuming packaged foods – such as crackers, chips, processed dips, sauces and sodas, for example – try cutting down on one or two items at a time, and over a while, gradually eliminate and cut down other items. Slowly replace these with fresh foods and healthier choices, so that your body has a chance to adapt without extreme cravings that often occur during sudden changes.

Quit Smoking and Reduce Alcohol

It's not easy to quit smoking or using recreational drugs, especially where there has been long-term use and the effects have already made an impact on your health. At some point, you'll begin to notice a difference in the way you feel and how your body changes over time. This includes chronic coughing related to respiratory conditions, shortness of breath, and a lack of energy. These changes may be subtle at first, and it may appear as though there is minimal damage or none at all, though smoking inevitably catches up with age and contributes to the development of cancer, premature aging and kidney damage. The more toxins we consume or add to our body, the more challenging it becomes for the kidneys to work efficiently, which eventually slows their ability to function.

For most people, quitting "cold turkey" or all at once is not an option, because of the withdrawal symptoms and increased chances of starting again. This method, however, can work if applied with a strong support system and a lot of determination, though it's not the best option for everyone. Reducing smoking on your own, or switching to e-cigarettes or a patch or medication, can help significantly over time. Setting goals of reduction until the point of quitting can be a beneficial way to visualize success and provide a sense of motivation. The following tips may also be useful for quitting smoking and other habit-forming substances:

Join a support group and talk to other people who relate to you. Share your struggles, ideas, and thoughts, which will help others as well as yourself during this process.

Track your progress on a calendar or in a notebook, either by pen and paper or on an application. This can serve as a motivator, as well as a means to display how you've done so far and where you can improve. For example, you may have reduced your smoking from ten to seven cigarettes per day, then increased to nine. This may indicate a slight change that can keep in mind to focus on reducing your intake further, from nine cigarettes to seven or six per day, and so on.

Be aware of stressors in your life that cause you to smoke or use substances. If these factors are avoidable, make every effort to minimize or stop them from impacting your life. This may include specific people, places, or situations that can "trigger" a craving or make you feel more likely to use than usual. If there are situations that you cannot avoid, such as family, work, or school-related situations, consult with a trusted friend or someone you can confide in who can be present with you during these instances.

Don't be afraid to ask for help. Many people cannot quit on their own without at least some assistance from others. Seeking the guidance and expertise of a counselor or medical professional to better yourself can be one of the most important decisions you make to improve the quality of your life.

Getting Active
One of the most important ways to keep fit and healthy is by staying active and engaging in regular exercise. Regular movement is key, and exercise is different for everyone, depending on their abilities and options available. Fortunately, there are unlimited ways to customize an exercise routine or plan that can suit any lifestyle, perhaps low impact to start, or if you're ready, engage in a more vigorous workout. For many people experiencing kidney disease, one of the major struggles is losing weight and living a sedentary life, where movement is generally minimal and exercise is generally not practiced. Smoking, eating processed foods, and not getting the required nutrition can further impair the body in such a way that exercise is seen as a hurdle and a challenge that is best avoided. Making lifestyle changes is not something that should be done all at once, but over a while – especially during the early stages of renal disease – so that the impact of the condition is minimized over time and becomes more manageable.

Where can you begin, if you haven't exercised at all or for a long period? For starters, don't sign up for a marathon or engage in any strenuous activities unless it is safe to do so. Start slow and take your time. Before taking on any new movements – whether it is minimal, low-impact walking or stretching, or a more moderate to the high-impact regimen – always talk to your doctor to rule out any impact this may have on other existing conditions, such as blood pressure and respiratory conditions, as well as your kidneys. Most, if not all, physicians will likely recommend exercise as part of the treatment plan but may advise beginning slowly if your body isn't used to exercise.

Simple techniques to introduce exercise into your life require a commitment. This can begin with a quick 15-minute walk or jog and a 10-or 15-minute stretch in the morning before starting your day. There are several easy, introductory techniques to consider, including the following:

Take a walk for 10 to 15 minutes each day, at least three or four days each week. If you find it difficult at first, due to cramping, respiratory issues, or other conditions, walk slowly and breathe deeply. Make sure you feel relaxed during your walks. Find a scenic path or area in your neighborhood that is pleasant and gives you something to enjoy, such as a beautiful sunset or forested park. Bring a bottle of water to keep yourself hydrated.

Stretch for five minutes once a day. This doesn't mean you need to do any intricate yoga poses or specific techniques. Moving your ankles, wrists, and arms in circles and standing every so often (if you sit often) and twisting your torso can help release stress and improve your blood flow, which lowers blood pressure and helps your body transport nutrients to areas in need of repair.

Practice breathing long, measured breaths. This will help prepare you for more endurance-based exercise, such as jogging, long walks, cycling, and swimming. Count to five on each inhale and exhale, and practice moving slowly as you breathe, to "sync" or coordinate your body's movements with your breathing. If you have difficulty with the respiratory system, take it slow and don't push yourself. If you feel weak or out of breath, stop immediately and try again later or the next day at a slower pace.

Start a beginner's yoga class and learn the fundamentals of various poses and stretches. It is helpful to arrive early and speak with the instructor, who can provide guidance on which modifications work best if needed. They may also be able to provide tips on how to approach certain poses or movements that can be challenging for beginners so that you feel more comfortable and knowledgeable before you start.

If you smoke, exercise will present more of a challenge on your lungs and respiratory function. Once you become accustomed to a beginner's level and become moderately active, you may notice it takes more effort, which requires an increase in lung capacity and oxygen. Smoking will eventually present a challenge, and where quitting can be a long-term and difficult goal in itself, make an effort to cut back as much as it takes to allow your body's movements and exercise continue. In time, you may find quitting becomes easier and more achievable than expected!

Once you get into a basic routine, there is a wide variety of individual and team activities to consider for your life. If you are a social person, joining a baseball team or badminton club

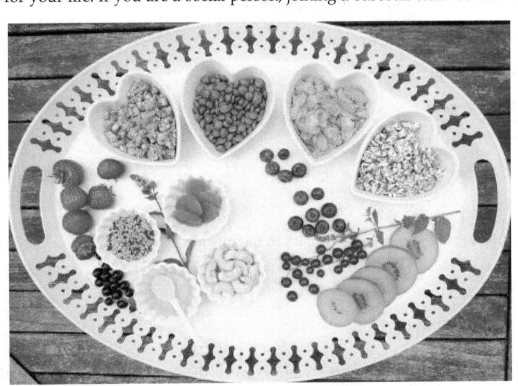

may be ideal. For more solitary options, consider swimming, cycling, or jogging. Many gyms and community centers provide monthly plans and may offer a free trial period to see if their facilities work for you. This is a great opportunity to try new classes and equipment to gauge how much you can achieve, even if in the early stages of exercise so that you can decide whether to pursue dance aerobics, spin classes and/or weight training. Some gyms will provide a free consultation with a personal trainer to set a simple plan towards weight loss and strength training goals.

Symptoms of kidney disease?

If kidney disease progresses, then the blood level of end products of metabolism increases; this in turn, is the cause of feeling unwell. Various health problems may occur, such as high blood pressure, anemia (anemia), bone disease, premature cardiovascular calcification, discoloration, and change in the composition and volume of urine.

As the disease progresses, the main symptoms can be:

- Weakness, a feeling of weakness

- Trouble sleeping

- Lack of appetite

- Dry skin, itchy skin

- Muscle cramps especially at night

- Swelling in the legs

- Swelling around the eyes, especially in the morning

The Causes of Kidney Failure

Renal disease, according to experts, requires early diagnosis and targeted treatment to prevent or delay both a condition of acute or chronic renal failure and the appearance of cardiovascular complications to which it is often associated.

In fact, hypertension and diabetes, not adequately controlled by drug therapy, prostatic hypertrophy, kidney stones or bulky tumors can promote onset as they reduce the normal flow of urine, increase the pressure inside the kidneys and limit functionality.

Or the kidney damage can be determined by inflammatory processes (pyelonephritis, glomerulonephritis) or by the formation of cysts inside the kidneys (polycystic kidney disease) or by the chronic use of some drugs, alcohol and drugs consumed in excess.

A fundamental role in alleviating the work of the already compromised kidneys is carried out by the diet which is, therefore, the first prevention. It must be studied with an expert nutritionist or a nephrologist in order to maintain or reach an ideal weight on the one hand and on the other to reduce the intake of sodium (salt), and the consequent control of blood pressure, and / or other substances (minerals), without creating malnutrition or nutritional deficiencies. Particular attention should also be paid to cholesterol, triglycerides and blood sugar levels.

Understanding what causes kidney failure goes a long way to deciding just what kind of treatment you should focus on. The most important factor that you should focus on is, of course, your diet. But as you focus on your diet, make sure that you are following your doctor's instructions, in the event of other complications. Let us look at a few of the common causes of kidney diseases.

Diabetes

We do know that diabetes is one of the leading causes of CKD. But we have yet to understand in detail why and how it can cause so much harm to the kidneys.

Time for a crash course in diabetes. What many may already know is that diabetes affects our body's insulin production rate. But what many may not know is the extent of damage that diabetes can cause to the kidneys.

High Blood Pressure

An important thing to remember here is that high blood pressure can be both a cause and symptom of CKD, similar to the case of diabetes.

So, what exactly is blood pressure? People often throw the term around, but they are unable to pinpoint exactly what happens when the pressure in the blood increases.

Autoimmune Diseases

IgA nephropathy and lupus are two examples of autoimmune diseases that can lead to kidney diseases. But just what exactly are autoimmune diseases?

They are conditions where your immune system perceives your body as a threat and begins to attack it.

We all know that the immune system is like the defense force of our body. It is responsible for guiding the soldiers of our body, known as white blood cells, or WBCs. The immune system is responsible for fighting against foreign materials, such as viruses and bacteria. When the system senses these foreign bodies, various fighter cells, including the WBCs, are deployed in order to combat the threat.

Typically, your immune system is a self-learning system. This means that it is capable of understanding the threat and memorizing its features, behaviors, and attack patterns. This is an important capability of the immune system since it allows the system to differentiate between our own cells and foreign cells. But when you have an autoimmune disease, your immune system suddenly considers certain parts of your body, such as your skin or joints, as foreign. It then proceeds to create antibodies that begin to

Diagnosis

There are two simple tests that your family doctor can prescribe to diagnose a kidney disease.

Blood test: glomerular filtration rate (GFR) and serum creatinine level. Creatinine is one of those end products of protein metabolism, the level of which in the blood depends on age, gender, muscle mass, nutrition, physical activity, the foods taken before taking the sample (for example, a lot of meat was eaten), and some drugs. Creatinine is removed from the body through the kidneys, and if the work of the kidneys slows down, the level of creatinine in the blood plasma increases. Determining the level of creatinine alone is not sufficient for the diagnosis of chronic kidney disease since its value begins to exceed the upper limit of the norm only when GFR is decreased by half. GFR is calculated using a formula that includes four parameters which are; the creatinine reading, age, gender, and race of the patient. GFR shows the level at which the kidneys can filter. In the case of chronic kidney disease, the GFR indicator indicates the stage of the severity of kidney disease.

Urine analysis: the content of albumin in the urine is determined; also, the values of albumin and creatinine in the urine are determined by each other. Albumin is a protein in the urine that usually enters the urine in minimal quantities. Even a small increase in the level of albumin in the urine in some people may be an early sign of incipient kidney disease, especially in those with diabetes and high blood pressure. In the case of normal kidney function, albumin in the urine should not be more than 3 mg/mmol (or 30 mg/g). If albumin excretion increases even more, then it already speaks of kidney disease.

Understand your Nutritional Needs

Potassium

Potassium is a naturally occurring mineral found in nearly all foods, in varying amounts. Our bodies need an amount of potassium to help with muscle activity as well as electrolyte balance and regulation of blood pressure. However, if potassium is in excess within the system and the kidneys can't expel it (due to renal disease), fluid retention and muscle spasms can occur.

Phosphorus

Phosphorus is a trace mineral found in a wide range of foods and especially dairy, meat, and eggs. It acts synergistic ally with calcium as well as Vitamin D to promote bone health. However, when there is damage in the kidneys, excess amounts of the mineral cannot be taken out and this can cause bone weakness.

Calories

When being on a renal diet, it is vital to give yourself the right number of calories to fuel your system. The exact number of calories you should consume daily depends on your age, gender, general health status and stage of renal disease. In most cases though, there are no strict limitations in the calorie intake, as long as you take them from proper sources that are low in sodium, potassium, and phosphorus. In general, doctors recommend a daily limit between 1800-2100 calories per day to keep weight within the normal range.

Protein

Protein is an essential nutrient that our systems need to develop and generate new connective tissue e.g. muscles, even during injuries. Protein also helps stop bleeding and supports the immune system fight infections. A healthy adult with no kidney disease would usually need 40-65 grams of protein per day.

However, in renal diet, protein consumption is a tricky subject as too much or too little can cause problems. Protein, when being metabolized by our systems also creates waste which is typically processed by the kidneys. But when kidneys are damaged or underperforming, as in the case of kidney disease that waste will stay in the system. This is why patients in more advanced CKD stages are advised to limit their protein consumption as well.

Fats

Our systems need fats and particularly good fats as a fuel source and for other metabolic cell functions. A diet rich in bad and Trans or saturated fats though can significantly raise the odds of developing heart problems, which often occur with the renal disease. This is why most physicians advise their renal patients to follow a diet that contains a decent amount of good fats and a meager amount of Trans (processed) or saturated fat.

Sodium

Sodium is an essential mineral that our bodies need to regulate fluid and electrolyte balance. It also plays a role in normal cell division in the muscles and nervous system. However, in kidney disease, sodium can quickly spike at higher than normal levels and the kidneys will be unable to expel it causing fluid accumulation as a side-effect. Those who also suffer from heart problems as well should limit its consumption as it may raise blood pressure.

Carbohydrates

Carbs act as a major and quick fuel source for the body's cells. When we consume carbs, our systems turn them into glucose and then into energy for "feeding" our body cells. Carbs are generally not restricted in the renal diet. Still, some types of carbs contain dietary fiber as well, which helps regulate normal colon function and protect blood vessels from damage.

Dietary Fiber

Fiber is an important element in our system that cannot be properly digested but plays a key role in the regulation of our bowel movements and blood cell protection. The fiber in the renal diet is generally encouraged as it helps loosen up the stools, relieve constipation and bloating and protect from colon damage. However, many patients don't get enough amounts of dietary fiber per day as many of them are high in potassium or phosphorus. Fortunately, there are some good dietary fiber sources for CKD patients that have lower amounts of these minerals compared to others.

Vitamins/Minerals

Our systems, according to medical research, need at least 13 vitamins and minerals to keep our cells fully active and healthy. Patients with renal disease though are more likely to be depleted by water-soluble vitamins like B-complex and Vitamin C, as a result, or limited fluid consumption. Therefore, supplementation with these vitamins along with a renal diet program should help cover any possible vitamin deficiencies. Supplementation of fat-soluble vitamins like vitamins A, K, and E may be avoided as they can quickly build up in the system and turn toxic.

Fluids

When you are in an advanced stage of renal disease, fluid can quickly build-up and lead to problems. While it is important to keep your system well hydrated, you should avoid minerals like potassium and sodium which can trigger further fluid build-up and cause a host of other symptoms.

Foods Recommended for your Health

There are many foods that work well within the renal diet, and once you see the available variety, it will not seem as restrictive or difficult to follow. The key is focusing on the foods with a high level of nutrients, which make it easier for the kidneys to process waste by not adding too much that the body needs to discard. Balance is a major factor in maintaining and improving long-term renal function.

Garlic

An excellent, vitamin-rich food for the immune system, garlic is a tasty substitute for salt in a variety of dishes. It acts as a significant source of vitamin C and B6, while aiding the kidneys in ridding the body of unwanted toxins. It's a great, healthy way to add flavor for skillet meals, pasta, soups, and stews.

Berries

All berries are considered a good renal diet food due to their high level of fiber, antioxidants, and delicious taste, making them an easy option to include as a light snack or as an ingredient in smoothies, salads, and light desserts. Just one handful of blueberries can provide almost one day's vitamin C requirement, as well as a boost of fiber, which is good for weight loss and maintenance.

Bell Peppers

Flavorful and easy to enjoy both raw and cooked, bell peppers offer a good source of vitamin C, vitamin A, and fiber. Along with other kidney-friendly foods, they make the detoxification process much easier while boosting your body's nutrient level to prevent further health conditions and reduce existing deficiencies.

Onions

This nutritious and tasty vegetable is excellent as a companion to garlic in many dishes, or on its own. Like garlic, onions can provide flavor as an alternative to salt, and provides a good source of vitamin C, vitamin B, manganese, and fiber, as well. Adding just one quarter or half of an onion is often enough for most meals, because of its strong, pungent flavor.

Macadamia Nuts

If you enjoy nuts and seeds as snacks, you many soon learn that many contain high amounts of phosphorus and should be avoided or limited as much as possible. Fortunately, macadamia nuts are an easier option to digest and process, as they contain much lower amounts of phosphorus and make an excellent substitute for other nuts. They are a good source of other nutrients, as well, such as vitamin B, copper, manganese, iron, and healthy fats.

Pineapple

Unlike other fruits that are high in potassium, pineapple is an option that can be enjoyed more often than bananas and kiwis. Citrus fruits are generally high in potassium as well, so if you find yourself craving an orange or grapefruit, choose pineapple instead. In addition to providing a high levels of vitamin B and fiber, pineapples can reduce inflammation thanks to an enzyme called brome lain.

Mushrooms

In general, mushrooms are a safe, healthy option for the renal diet, especially the shiitake variety, which are high in nutrients such as selenium, vitamin B, and manganese. They contain a moderate amount of plant-based protein, which is easier for your body to digest and use than animal proteins. Shiitake and Portobello mushrooms are often used in vegan diets as a meat substitute, due to their texture and pleasant flavor.

Foods that are Toxic and Harmful to Health

Eating restrictions might be different depending upon your level of kidney disease. If you are in the early stages of kidney disease, you may have different restrictions as compared to those who are at the end-stage renal disease, or kidney failure. In contrast to this, people with an end-stage renal disease requiring dialysis will face different eating restrictions. Let's discuss some of the foods to avoid while being on the renal diet.

Dark-Colored Colas contain calories, sugar, phosphorus, etc. They contain phosphorus to enhance flavor, increase its life and avoid discoloration. Which can be found in a product's ingredient list. This addition of phosphorus varies depending on the type of cola. Mostly, the dark-colored colas contain 50–100 mg in a 200-ml serving. Therefore, dark colas should be avoided on a renal diet.

Canned Foods including soups, vegetables, and beans, are low in cost but contain high amounts of sodium due to the addition of salt to increase its life. Due to this amount of sodium inclusion in canned goods, it is better that people with kidney disease should avoid consumption. Opt for lower-sodium content with the label "no salt added". One more way is to drain or rinse canned foods, such as canned beans and tuna, could decrease the sodium content by 33–80%, depending on the product.

Brown Rice is a whole grain containing a higher concentration of potassium and phosphorus than its white rice counterpart. One cup already cooked brown rice possess about 150 mg of phosphorus and 154 mg of potassium, whereas, one cup of already cooked white rice has an amount of about 69 mg of phosphorus and 54 mg of potassium. Bulgur, buckwheat, pearled barley and couscous are equally beneficial, low-phosphorus options and might be a good alternative instead of brown rice.

Bananas are high potassium content, low in sodium, and provides 422 mg of potassium per banana. It might disturb your daily balanced potassium intake to 2,000 mg if a banana is a daily staple.

Whole-Wheat Bread may harm individuals with kidney disease. But for healthy individuals, it is recommended over refined, white flour bread. White bread is recommended instead of whole-wheat varieties for individuals with kidney disease just because it has phosphorus and potassium. If you add more bran and whole grains in the bread, then the amount of phosphorus and potassium contents goes higher.

Oranges and Orange Juice are enriched with vitamin C content and potassium. 184 grams provides 333 mg of potassium and 473 mg of potassium in one cup of orange juice. With these calculations, oranges and orange juice must be avoided or used in a limited amount while being on a renal diet.

Potatoes and sweet potatoes, being, the potassium-rich vegetables with 156 g contains 610 mg of potassium, whereas 114 g contains 541 mg of potassium which is relatively high. Some of the high-potassium foods, likewise potatoes and sweet potatoes, could also be soaked or leached to lessen the concentration of potassium contents. Cut them into small and thin pieces and boil those for at least 10 minutes can reduce the potassium content by about 50%. Potatoes which are soaked in a wide pot of water for as low as four hours before cooking could possess even less potassium content than those not soaked before cooking. This is known as "potassium leaching," or the "double cook Direction."

If you are suffering from or living with kidney disease, reducing your potassium, phosphorus and sodium intake is an essential aspect of managing and tackling the disease. The foods with high-potassium, high-sodium, and high-phosphorus content listed above should always be limited or avoided. These restrictions and nutrients intakes may differ depending on the level of damage to your kidneys. Following a renal diet might be a daunting procedure and a restrictive one most of the times. But, working with your physician and nutrition specialist and a renal dietitian can assist you to formulate a renal diet specific to your individual needs.

How to Manage the Renal Diet When You Are Diabetic

Patients who struggle from kidney health issues, going through kidney dialysis and have renal impairments need to not only go through medical treatment but also change their eating habit, lifestyle to make the situation better. Many researches have been done on this, and the conclusion is food has a lot to do with how your kidney functions and its overall health.

The first thing to changing your lifestyle is knowing about how your kidney functions and how different food can trigger different reactions in the kidney function. There are certain nutrients that affect your kidney directly. Nutrients like sodium, protein, phosphate, and potassium are the risky ones. You do not have to omit them altogether from your diet, but you need to limit or minimize their intake as much as possible. You cannot leave out essential nutrient like protein from your diet, but you need to count how much protein you are having per day. This is essential in order to keep balance in your muscles and maintaining a good functioning kidney.

A vast change in kidney patients is measuring how much fluid they are drinking. This is a crucial change in every kidney patient, and you must adapt to this new eating habit. Too much water or any other form of liquid can disrupt your kidney function. How much fluid you can consume depends on the condition of your kidney. Most people assign separate bottles for them so that they can measure how much they have drunk and how much more they can drink throughout the day.

Adopt a Healthy Lifestyle To Reduce The Occurrence Of Kidney Disease.

Once a kidney is damaged there is no one-time solution or magic to undo all the damage. It requires constant management and a whole new lifestyle to provide a healthy environment for your kidneys. For healthy kidneys, you just need to keep the following in mind:

Upgrade your vegetable intake to 5–9 vegetables per day.

Reduce the salt intake in your diet.

Cut down the overall protein intake.

Remove all the triggers of heart diseases, like fats and sugar, from your diet.

Do not consume pesticides and other environmental contaminants.

Try to consume fresh food; homemade is the best.

Avoid using food additives, as they contain high amounts of potassium, sodium, and phosphorous.

Drink lots of sodium-free drinks, especially water.

Choose to be more active and exercise regularly.

Do not smoke to avoid toxicity.

Obesity can create a greater risk of kidney diseases, so control your weight.

Do not take painkillers excessively, such as Ibuprofen, as they can also damage your kidneys.

Tips and Advice for Those with Kidney Disease

Tips on controlling your phosphorous

Here is what you should do to maintain a balanced level of phosphorous:

- Limit the consumption of foods like poultry, meats, fish and dairy
- Limit the intake of certain dairy products like yogurt and cheese; you should not exceed 4 oz. Per serving
- Avoid black beans, lima beans, red beans, garbanzo beans, white beans and black-eyed peas.
- Avoid unrefined, whole and dark grains.
- Stay away from refrigerator dough
- Avoid dried fruits and vegetables
- Avoid chocolate
- Avoid sodas that are dark-colored
- Make sure to take your phosphate folders with your snacks and meals.
- The renal diet limits the intake of phosphorus to 1000mg per day

Tips on Controlling your Protein

Make sure to consume high-quality proteins. Eat about 7 to 8 oz. of protein per day. Pork, beef, turkey, veal; chicken and eggs have high amounts of protein.

Tips on Controlling your Fluid Intake

- Use 1 cup or glass in order to divide your fluid intake per day. You can also write a record of your fluid intake.
- Always avoid any type of salty food and never add extra salt to your meals.
- Avoid processed meats, fast foods and canned foods
- You can add lemon juice to the water you want to drink instead
- You can clean your mouth with a mouthwash from time to time
- Avoid overheating
- Maintain your blood sugar at a balanced level

Eating Out

Look out for small or half portions and ask your server for your foods to be cooked without extra salt, butter or sauce. Avoid fried foods, instead, embrace poached or grilled food. If you know, you are going out to eat, plan ahead. Look at the restaurant menu beforehand online.

Eating at social gatherings (such as birthdays, weddings, picnics, and barbecues)

1. Don't go hungry: Have a snack before you leave the house.

2. Avoid high-sodium foods: Avoid foods such as hot dogs or sausages. Choose lower-sodium foods such as chicken and hamburgers.

3. Limit alcohol: Speak with your physician first about drinking alcohol.

4. Plan ahead: Plan your menus.

Seafood

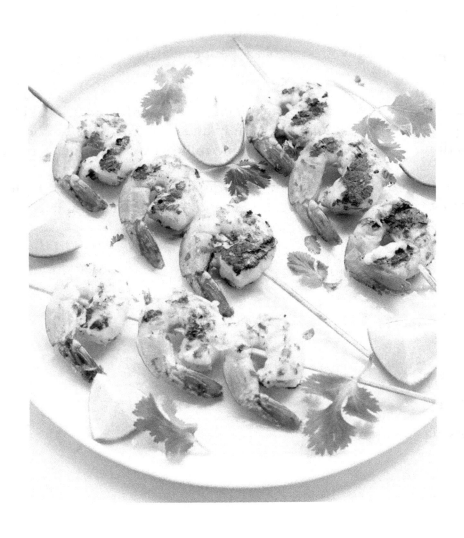

Corn and Shrimp Quiche

Preparation Time: 15 minutes

Cooking Time: 50 minutes

Servings: 6

Ingredients:

- 1 cup of small cooked shrimp
- 1½ cups of frozen corn, thawed and drained
- ¾ cup of shredded sharp Colby cheese
- 5 large eggs, beaten
- 1 cup of unsweetened almond milk
- Pinch salt
- 1/8 teaspoon of freshly ground black pepper

Directions:

1. Preheat the oven to 350°F. Spray a 9-inch pie pan with nonstick baking spray.
2. In the prepared pan, combine the shrimp and corn. Sprinkle the cheese over the top.
3. In a medium bowl, beat the eggs, almond milk, salt, and pepper. Gently pour into the pan.
4. Bake for 45 to 55 minutes or until the quiche is puffed, set to the touch, and light golden brown on top. Make sure it is cool enough before cutting into wedges to serve.

Nutrition:

Calories: 198

Total fat: 10g

Saturated fat: 4g

Sodium: 238mg

Phosphorus: 260mg

Potassium: 261mg

Carbohydrates: 9g

Fiber: 1g

Protein: 20g

Sugar: 2g

Ginger Shrimp with Snow Peas

Preparation Time: 20 minutes
Cooking Time: 12 minutes
Servings: 4
Ingredients:

- 2 tablespoons of extra-virgin olive oil
- 1 tablespoon of minced peeled fresh ginger
- 2 cups of snow peas
- 1½ cups of frozen baby peas
- 3 tablespoons of water
- 1 pound of medium shrimp, shelled and deveined
- 2 tablespoons of low-sodium soy sauce
- 1/8 teaspoon of freshly ground black pepper

Directions:

1. Using a large wok, heat the olive oil over medium heat.
2. Add the ginger and stir-fry for 1 to 2 minutes, until the ginger is fragrant.
3. Add the snow peas and stir-fry for 2 to 3 minutes, until they are tender-crisp.
4. Add the baby peas and the water and stir. Cover the wok and steam for 2 to 3 minutes or until the vegetables are tender.
5. Stir in the shrimp and stir-fry for 3 to 4 minutes, or until the shrimp have curled and turned pink.
6. Add the soy sauce and pepper; stir and serve.

Nutrition:
Calories: 237
Total fat: 7g
Saturated fat: 1g
Sodium: 469mg
Phosphorus: 350mg
Potassium: 504mg
Carbohydrates: 12g
Fiber: 4g
Protein: 32g
Sugar: 5g

Roasted Cod with Plums

Preparation Time: 10 minutes

Cooking Time: 20 minutes

Servings: 4

Ingredients:

- 6 red plums, halved and pitted
- 1½ pounds cod fillets
- 3 tablespoons extra-virgin olive oil
- 2 tablespoons freshly squeezed lemon juice
- ½ teaspoon dried thyme leaves
- 1/8 teaspoon salt
- 1/8 teaspoon freshly ground black pepper
- ¾ cup plain whole-milk yogurt, for serving

Directions:

1. Preheat the oven to 375°F. Line a baking sheet with parchment paper.
2. Arrange the plums, cut-side up, along with the fish on the prepared baking sheet. Put the olive oil and lemon juice and sprinkle with the thyme, salt, and pepper.
3. Roast for 15 to 20 minutes or until the fish flakes when tested with a fork and the plums are tender.
4. Serve with the yogurt.

Nutrition:

Calories: 230

Total fat: 9g

Saturated fat: 2g

Sodium: 154mg

Phosphorus: 197mg

Potassium: 437mg

Carbohydrates: 10g

Fiber: 1g

Protein: 27g

Sugar: 8g

Family Hit Curry

Preparation Time: 10 minutes
Cooking Time: 21 minutes
Servings: 8
Ingredients:

- 1½ tbsp. of canola oil
- 1 finely chopped onion
- 1 tsp. of minced fresh ginger
- 3 minced garlic cloves
- 1 tbsp. of curry paste
- 2 cups of fat-free plain Greek yogurt
- ¼ cup of water
- 1 tsp. of sugar
- 1 pound of cubed cod fillets
- 1 pound of peeled and deveined prawns
- Pinch of salt
- Freshly ground black pepper, to taste
- 2 tbsp. of fresh lemon juice
- ¼ cup of chopped fresh cilantro leaves

Directions:

1. In a large pan, heat oil on medium heat. Add onion and sauté for about 4–5 minutes.
2. Add ginger, garlic, and curry paste and sauté for about 1 minute.
3. Stir in yogurt, water, and sugar and bring to a boil on high heat.
4. Reduce the heat to medium-low. Simmer for about 5 minutes.
5. Stir in seafood and cook for about 10 minutes or till desired thickness.
6. Stir in salt, black pepper, lemon juice, and cilantro and remove from heat.
7. Serve hot.

Nutrition:
Calories: 191
Fat: 5.3g
Carbs: 5g
Protein: 29.2g
Fiber: 0g
Potassium: 270mg
Sodium: 199mg

Homemade Tuna Nicoise

Preparation Time: 5 minutes
Cooking Time: 10 minutes
Servings: 2
Ingredients:

- 1 egg
- ½ cup of green beans
- ¼ sliced cucumber
- 1 lemon's juice
- 1 tsp. of black pepper
- ¼ sliced red onion
- 1 tbsp. of olive oil
- 1 tbsp. of capers
- 4 oz. of drained canned tuna
- 4 iceberg lettuce leaves
- 1 tsp. of chopped fresh cilantro

Directions:

1. Prepare the salad by washing and slicing the lettuce, cucumber, and onion.
2. Add to a salad bowl.
3. Mix 1 tbsp. of oil with the lemon juice, cilantro, and capers for a salad dressing. Set aside.
4. Boil a pan of water on high heat, then lower to simmer and add the egg for 6 minutes. (Steam the green beans over the same pan in a steamer/colander for the 6 minutes.)
5. Remove the egg and rinse under cold water.
6. Peel before slicing in half.
7. Mix the tuna, salad, and dressing in a salad bowl.
8. Toss to coat.
9. Top with the egg and serve with a sprinkle of black pepper.

Nutrition:
Calories: 199
Protein: 19g
Carbs: 7g
Fat: 8g
Sodium: 466mg
Potassium: 251mg
Phosphorus: 211mg

Cajun Crab

Preparation Time: 10 minutes

Cooking Time: 10 minutes

Servings: 2

Ingredients:

- 1 lemon, fresh and quartered
- 3 tablespoons of Cajun seasoning
- 2 bay leaves
- 4 snow crab legs, precooked and defrosted
- Golden ghee

Directions:

1. Fill a large pot with salted water about halfway.
2. Bring the water to a boil.
3. Squeeze lemon juice into a pot and toss in remaining lemon quarters.
4. Add bay leaves and Cajun seasoning.
5. Then season for 1 minute.
6. Add crab legs and boil for 8 minutes (make sure to keep them submerged the whole time).
7. Melt ghee in the microwave and use as a dipping sauce, enjoy!

Nutrition:

Calories: 643

Fat: 51g

Carbohydrates: 3g

Protein: 41g

Creamy Crab Soup

Preparation Time: 10 minutes

Cooking Time: 15–20 minutes

Servings: 7–8

Ingredients:

- 1 tbsp. of low salt butter
- 1 cup of white onion, chopped
- ½ pound of fresh crab meat
- 4 cups of low-salt chicken broth
- 1 cup of soy or vegetable cream
- 2 tbsp. of cornstarch
- 1/8 tsp. of dill
- Kosher pepper

Directions:

1. Melt the butter in a large pan over medium heat.
2. Add the onion to the pot and sauté until transparent, for around 3 minutes.
3. Add the crab meat to the mix and cook for another couple of minutes.
4. Add the chicken broth to the pan mix and bring to a boil.
5. Mix the vegetable or soy cream with the cornstarch and whisk to combine well. Add to the soup and increase the heat to medium-high.
6. Add the dill and pepper and stir frequently until soup comes to a boil.
7. Serve hot.

Nutrition:

Calories: 89

Carbohydrate: 10g

Protein: 7g

Sodium: 228mg

Potassium: 237mg

Phosphorus: 83mg

Dietary Fiber: 0.3g

Fat: 3.7g

Spicy Lime Shrimp

Preparation Time: 10 minutes

Cooking Time: 5 minutes

Servings: 4–5

Ingredients:

- 32 large shrimp, peeled and deveined
- ¼ cup of lime juice
- 1 garlic clove, minced
- 1 green onion, sliced
- 3 tbsp. of red bell pepper, diced
- 2 tbsp. of fresh cilantro, chopped
- 1 tsp. of jalapeno chili, minced
- 1/8 tsp. of salt
- 1 big cucumber, sliced

Directions:

1. To make your dressing, combine the lime juice, green onion, jalapeno chili, cilantro, garlic, and oil or salt in a mixing bowl.
2. In a separate mixing bowl, add the shrimps with 3 tbsp of the lime juice marinade. Cover and let in the fridge for 40 minutes.
3. Turn on your oven's broiler. Discard the shrimp from the lime marinade and broil for around 3-4 minutes in total or 2 minutes on each side.
4. Take off the heat and pour the remaining marinade on top.
5. Place over the cucumber slices and serve cold.

Nutrition:

Calories: 132

Carbohydrate: 3g

Protein: 12g

Sodium: 149mg

Potassium: 202mg

Phosphorus: 128mg

Dietary Fiber: 0.6g

Fat: 8g

Seafood Casserole

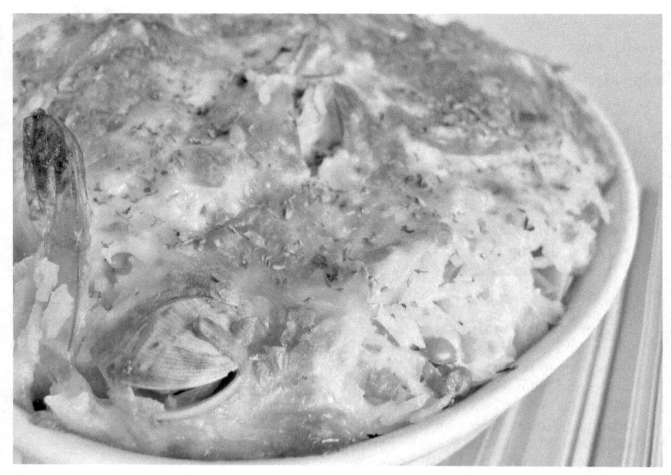

Preparation Time: 20 minutes

Cooking Time: 45 minutes

Servings: 6

Ingredients:

- 2 cups eggplant—peeled and diced into 1-inch pieces
- Butter, for greasing the baking sheet
- 1 tbsp. of olive oil
- ½ sweet onion, chopped
- 1 tsp. of minced garlic
- 1 stalk of celery, chopped
- ½ red bell pepper, boiled and chopped

- 3 tbsps. of freshly squeezed lemon juice
- 1 tsp. of hot sauce
- ¼ tsp. of creole seasoning mix
- ½ cup of uncooked white rice
- 1 large egg
- 4 ounces of cooked shrimp
- 6 ounces of queen crab meat

Directions:
1. Preheat the oven to 350°F.
2. Boil the eggplant in a saucepan for 5 minutes. Drain and set aside.
3. Grease a 9-by-13-inch baking sheet with butter and set aside.
4. Heat the olive oil in a large skillet over medium heat.
5. Sauté the garlic, onion, celery, and bell pepper for 4 minutes or until tender.
6. Add the sautéed vegetables to the eggplant, along with the lemon juice, hot sauce, seasoning, rice, and egg.
7. Stir to combine.
8. Fold in the shrimp and crab meat.
9. Spoon the casserole mixture into the casserole dish, patting down the top.
10.   Bake for 25 to 30 minutes or until casserole is heated through and rice is tender.
11.   Serve warm.

Nutrition:

Calories: 118

Fat: 4g

Carb: 9g

Phosphorus: 102mg

Potassium: 199mg

Sodium: 235mg

Protein: 12g

Tilapia Ceviche

Preparation Time: 15 minutes
Cooking Time: 5 minutes
Servings: 1 cup with 6 crackers
Ingredients:

- 1½ pounds of fresh tilapia fillets
- 1 cup of red onion
- ½ cup of red bell pepper
- ¼ cup of cilantro
- 1 cup of pineapple
- 2 tablespoons of canola oil
- ¼ teaspoon of black pepper
- 1¼ cups of fresh lime juice
- 48 saltine crackers with unsalted tops

Directions:

1. Chop the onion, bell pepper, and cilantro. Also, dice the pineapple, and cube the tilapia into small chunks.
2. Broil tilapia cubes over high heat for about 3 minutes on each side.
3. Cool the tilapia for about 5 minutes, then pour the fresh lime juice on top of it, mixing properly. Ensure all tilapia pieces are coated completely with the lime juice.
4. Combine and mix the bell pepper, onion, pineapple, cilantro, black pepper, and the canola oil with the broiled tilapia mixture.
5. Cover and refrigerate to marinate for about 2 hours.
6. Use six saltine crackers with the unsalted tops for each serving.

Nutrition:
Calories: 220
Protein: 19g
Carbohydrates: 20g
Fat: 7g
Cholesterol: 36mg
Sodium: 168mg
Potassium: 374mg
Phosphorus: 162mg
Fiber: 1.3g

Fish Tacos

Preparation Time: 10 minutes

Cooking Time: 35 minutes

Servings: 6

Ingredients:

- 1½ cup of cabbage
- ½ cup of red onion
- ½ bunch of cilantro
- 1 garlic clove
- 2 limes
- 1 pound of cod fillets
- ½ teaspoon of ground cumin
- ½ teaspoon of chili powder
- ¼ teaspoon of black pepper
- 1 tablespoon of olive oil
- ½ cup of mayonnaise
- ¼ cup of sour cream
- 2 tablespoons of milk
- 12 (6-inch) corn tortillas

Directions:

1. Shred the cabbage, chop the onion and cilantro, and mince the garlic. Set aside.
2. Use a dish to place in the fish fillets, then squeeze half a lime juice over the fish. Sprinkle the fish fillets with the minced garlic, cumin, black pepper, chili powder, and olive oil. Turn the fish filets to coat with the marinade, then refrigerate for about 15 to 30 minutes.
3. Prepare salsa Blanca by mixing the mayonnaise, milk, sour cream, and the other half of the lime juice. Stir to combine, then place in the refrigerator to chill.
4. Broil in oven, and cover the broiler pan with aluminum foil. Broil the coated fish fillets for about 10 minutes or until the flesh becomes opaque and white and flakes easily. Remove from the oven, slightly cool, and then flake the fish into bigger pieces.
5. Heat the corn tortillas in a pan, one at a time until it becomes soft and warm, then wrap in a dish towel to keep them warm.
6. To assemble the tacos, place a piece of the fish on the tortilla, topping with the salsa blanca, cabbage, cilantro, red onion, and the lime wedges.
7. Serve with hot sauce if you desire.

Nutrition:

Calories: 363

Protein: 18g

Carbohydrates: 30g

Fat: 19g

Cholesterol: 40mg

Sodium: 194mg

Potassium: 507mg

Phosphorus: 327mg

Fiber: 4.3g

Jambalaya

Preparation Time: 10 minutes

Cooking Time: 1 hour and 15 minutes

Servings: 12

Ingredients:

- 2 cups of onion
- 1 cup of bell pepper
- 2 garlic cloves
- 2 cups of uncooked converted brown rice
- ½ teaspoon of black pepper
- 8 ounces of canned low-sodium tomato sauce
- 2 cups of low-sodium beef broth
- 2 pounds of raw shrimp
- ½ cup of unsalted margarine

Directions:

1. Preheat oven to 350°F.
2. Chop the onion, bell pepper, garlic, then peel the shrimp.
3. Combine and mix all the ingredients in a large bowl except the margarine.
4. Pour into a 9 x 13-inch baking sheet and evenly spread out.
5. Slice the margarine, placing over the top of the ingredients.
6. Cover with foil or lid, and bake for about 1 hr. 15 minutes.
7. Serve hot.

Nutrition:

Calories: 294

Protein: 20g

Carbohydrates: 31g

Fat: 10g

Cholesterol: 137mg

Sodium: 186mg

Potassium: 300mg

Phosphorus: 197mg

Fiber: 0.8g

Asparagus Shrimp Linguini

Preparation Time: 10 minutes

Cooking Time: 35 minutes

Servings: 1 ½ cup

Ingredients:

- 8 ounces of uncooked linguini
- 1 tablespoon of olive oil
- 1¾ cups of asparagus
- ½ cup of unsalted butter
- 2 garlic cloves
- 3 ounces of cream cheese
- 2 tablespoons of fresh parsley
- ¾ teaspoon of dried basil
- 2/3 cup of dry white wine
- ½ pound of peeled and cooked shrimp

Directions:

1. Preheat oven to 350°F.
2. Cook the linguini in boiling water until it becomes tender, then drain.
3. Place the asparagus on a baking sheet, then spread two tablespoons of oil over the asparagus. Bake for about 7 to 8 minutes or until it is tender.
4. Remove baked asparagus from the oven and place it on a plate. Cut the asparagus into pieces of medium-sized once cooled.
5. Mince the garlic and chop the parsley.
6. Melt ½ cup of butter in a large skillet with the minced garlic.
7. Stir in the cream cheese, mixing as it melts.
8. Stir in the parsley and basil, then simmer for about 5 minutes. Mix either in boiling water or dry white wine, stirring until the sauce becomes smooth.
9. Add the cooked shrimp and asparagus, then stir and heat until it is evenly warm.
10. Toss the cooked pasta with the sauce and serve.

Nutrition:

Calories: 544

Protein: 21g

Carbohydrates: 43g

Fat: 32g

Cholesterol: 188mg

Sodium: 170mg

Potassium: 402mg

Phosphorus: 225mg

Fiber: 2.4g

Tuna Noodle Casserole

Preparation Time: 10 minutes

Cooking Time: 35 minutes

Servings: 2

Ingredients:

- 2 ounces of wide uncooked egg noodles
- 5 ounces of canned tuna in water
- ½ cup of sour cream
- ¼ cup of cottage cheese
- ½ cup of fresh sliced mushrooms
- ½ cup of frozen green peas
- 1 tablespoon of unsalted butter
- ¼ cup of unseasoned bread crumbs

Directions:

1. Preheat oven to 350°F.

2. Boil egg noodles based on the package instructions and drain. Also, drain and flake the tuna.

3. Combine and mix the sour cream, cottage cheese, mushrooms, tuna, and peas in a medium bowl.

4. Stir the drained noodle into the tuna mixture, and place it in a small casserole dish that has been sprayed with a non-stick cooking spray.

5. Melt butter, stir into the bread crumbs, then sprinkle over the mixture of noodles in step 4.

6. Bake for about 20 to 25 minutes or until the bread crumbs start to brown.

7. Divide into two and serve.

Nutrition:

Calories: 415

Protein: 22g

Carbohydrates: 39g

Fat: 19g

Cholesterol: 88mg

Sodium: 266mg

Potassium: 400mg

Phosphorus: 306mg

Fiber: 3.2g

Oven-Fried Southern Style Catfish

Preparation Time: 10 minutes
Cooking Time: 35 minutes
Servings: 4
Ingredients:

- 1 egg white
- ½ cup of all-purpose flour
- ¼ cup of cornmeal
- ¼ cup of panko bread crumbs
- 1 teaspoon of salt-free Cajun seasoning
- 1 pound of catfish fillets

Directions:

1. Heat oven to 450°F.
2. Use cooking spray to spray a non-stick baking sheet.
3. Using a bowl, beat the egg white until very soft peaks are formed. Don't over-beat.
4. Use a sheet of wax paper and place the flour over it.
5. Use a different sheet of wax paper to combine and mix the cornmeal, panko, and the Cajun seasoning.
6. Cut the catfish fillet into four pieces, then dip the fish in the flour, shaking off the excess.
7. Dip coated fish in the egg white, rolling into the cornmeal mixture.
8. Place the fish on the baking pan. Repeat with the remaining fish fillets.
9. Use cooking spray to spray over the fish fillets. Bake for about 10 to 12 minutes or until the sides of the fillets become browned and crisp.

Nutrition:
Calories: 250
Protein: 22g
Carbohydrates: 19g
Fat: 10g
Cholesterol: 53mg
Sodium: 124mg
Potassium: 401mg
Phosphorus: 262mg
Fiber: 1.2g

Cilantro-Lime Cod

Preparation Time: 10 minutes

Cooking Time: 35 minutes

Servings: 4

Ingredients:

- ½ cup of mayonnaise
- ½ cup of fresh chopped cilantro
- 2 tablespoon of lime juice
- 1 pound of cod fillets

Directions:

1. Combine and mix the mayonnaise, cilantro, and lime juice in a medium bowl, remove ¼ cup to another bowl and put aside. To be served as fish sauce.
2. Spread the remaining mayonnaise mixture over the cod fillets.
3. Use cooking spray to spray a large skillet, then heat over medium-high heat.
4. Place in the cod fillets, and cook for about 8 minutes or until the fish becomes firm and moist, turning just once.
5. Serve with the ¼ cilantro-lime sauce.

Nutrition:

Calories: 292

Protein: 20g

Carbohydrates: 1g

Fat: 23g

Cholesterol: 57mg

Sodium: 228mg

Potassium: 237mg

Phosphorus: 128mg

Calcium: 14mg

Shrimp Quesadilla

Preparation Time: 15 minutes

Cooking Time: 10 minutes

Servings: 2

Ingredients:

- 5 ounces of raw shrimp
- 2 tablespoons of cilantro
- 1 tablespoon of lemon juice
- ¼ teaspoon of ground cumin
- 1/8 teaspoon of cayenne pepper
- 2 flour burrito-sized tortillas
- 2 tablespoons of sour cream
- 4 teaspoons of salsa
- 2 tablespoons of shredded jalapeno cheddar cheese

Directions:

1. Peel the shrimp, rinse, and then cut into pieces of bite-size. Dice the cilantro.
2. Use a zip-lock bag to combine and mix the cilantro, lemon juice, cumin, and cayenne pepper to make the marinade. Add the pieces of shrimp and put aside to marinate for about 5 minutes.
3. Heat a skillet over medium heat and add the shrimp with the marinade. Stir-fry for about 1 to 2 minutes or until the shrimp is orange in color. Remove the skillet from heat and spoon out the shrimp, leaving marinade.
4. Add the sour cream to the skillet with the leftover marinade. Stir to mix.
5. Use a large skillet or microwave to heat the tortillas, then spread two teaspoons of salsa over each tortilla. Top with ½ of the shrimp mixture, sprinkling with one tablespoon of cheddar cheese.
6. Spoon out one tablespoon of the sour cream mixture from step 4 on top of the shrimp, fold the tortilla into half, turning over in skillet to heat, then remove from the pan. Repeat the same process with the second tortilla and with the remaining shrimp, cheese, and marinade.
7. Cut each of the tortillas into four pieces, and serve.

Nutrition:

Calories: 318

Protein: 20g

Carbohydrates: 26g

Fat: 15g

Cholesterol: 118mg

Sodium: 398mg

Potassium: 276mg

Phosphorus: 243mg

Fiber: 1.2g

Maryland Crab Cakes

Preparation Time: 5 minutes
Cooking Time: 15 minutes
Servings: 6
Ingredients:

- 1 pound of lump crab meat
- 1 slice of white bread
- 1 tablespoon of mayonnaise
- 1 teaspoon of yellow mustard
- 1 teaspoon of 30%-less-sodium Old Bay seasoning
- 1 tablespoon of fresh parsley
- 1/8 teaspoon of cayenne pepper
- 1 large egg
- 2 tablespoons of olive oil

Directions:

1. Pick through the crab meat in a medium bowl, removing any shell pieces.
2. Cut the slice of bread into cubes.
3. Add in all the ingredients except the olive oil. Mix slightly until all the ingredients are combined. Don't over mix.
4. Portion out six crab cakes using 1/3cup, with each portion being ¾ inch thick. Store in the refrigerator for one hour.
5. Heat oil or cooking spray in a heavy skillet and fry both sides of the crab for 5 minutes each or until it becomes brown.

Nutrition:
Calories: 158
Protein: 17g
Carbohydrates: 2g
Fat: 9g
Cholesterol: 112mg
Sodium: 337mg
Potassium: 268mg
Phosphorus: 177mg
Fiber: 0.3g

Citrus Grilled Glazed Salmon

Preparation Time: 10 minutes
Cooking Time: 20 minutes
Servings: 6
Ingredients:

- 2 garlic cloves
- 1½ tablespoons of lemon juice
- 2 tablespoons of olive oil
- 1 tablespoon of unsalted butter
- 1 tablespoon of Dijon mustard
- 2 dashes of cayenne pepper
- 1 teaspoon of dried basil leaves
- 1 teaspoon of dried dill
- 1 tablespoon of capers
- 24 ounces of salmon filet

Directions:

1. Crush the garlic.
2. Combine all ingredients in a small saucepan, excluding the salmon, heat to a boil, then reduce the heat to low — Cook for about 5 minutes.
3. Preheat grill, then place the salmon with its skin side down on a sheet of foil that is a little bigger than the fish. Fold up the edges so that the sauce remains with the salmon on the grill. Place on top of the grill, the foil, and fish, then top the salmon with the sauce mixture from step 2.
4. Cover grill and cook for about 12 minutes or until the salmon has cooked (don't flip the salmon).
5. Cut the salmon into six servings.

Nutrition:
Calories: 294
Protein: 23g
Carbohydrates: 1g
Fat: 22g
Cholesterol: 68mg
Sodium: 190mg
Potassium: 439mg
Phosphorus: 280mg
Fiber: 0.2g

Omega-3 Rich Salmon

Preparation Time: 10 minutes

Cooking Time: 20-25 minutes

Servings: 2

Ingredients:

- 2 (4-ounce) skinless, boneless salmon fillets
- 2 tbsp. of fresh lemon juice
- 1 tbsp. of olive oil
- ¼ tsp. of crushed dried oregano
- Pinch of salt
- Freshly ground black pepper, to taste

Directions:

1. Preheat the oven to 425°F. Line a baking sheet with parchment paper.
2. Place the salmon fillets onto the prepared baking sheet.
3. Drizzle with lemon juice and oil evenly and sprinkle with oregano, salt, and black pepper.
4. Bake for about 20–25 minutes.
5. Serve hot.

Nutrition:

Calories: 265

Fat: 19.2g

Carbs: 0.5g

Protein: 22.3g

Fiber: 0g

Potassium: 23mg

Sodium: 146mg

Smoothies

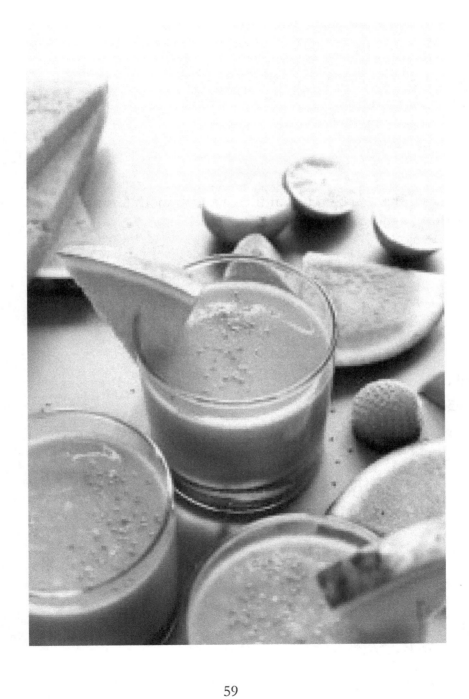

Sunny Pineapple Breakfast Smoothie

Preparation Time: 5 minutes

Cooking Time: 1 minute

Servings: 1

Ingredients:

- ½ cup of frozen pineapple chunks
- 2/3 cup of almond milk
- ½ tsp. of ginger powder
- 1 tbsp. of agave syrup

Directions:

1. Blend everything in a blender until nice and smooth (around 30 seconds).
2. Transfer into a tall glass or Mason jar.
3. Serve and enjoy.

Nutrition:

Calories: 186

Carbohydrate: 43.7g

Protein: 2.28g

Sodium: 130mg

Potassium: 135mg

Phosphorus: 18mg

Dietary Fiber: 2.4g

Fat: 2.3g

Blueberry Burst Smoothie

Preparation Time: 5 minutes

Cooking Time: 0 minute

Servings: 2

Ingredients:

- 1 cup of blueberries
- 1 cup of chopped collard greens
- 1 cup of Homemade Rice Milk or unsweetened store-bought rice milk
- 1 tablespoon of almond butter
- 3 ice cubes

Directions:

1. In a blender, combine the blueberries, collard greens, milk, almond butter, and ice cubes.
2. Process until smooth, and serve.

Nutrition tip: Collard greens are a nutrient-dense food loaded with anticarcinogenic, antiviral, antibiotic, and antioxidant properties. Because collard greens are much lower in potassium than kale, they are a great substitute in recipes that call for its cruciferous cousin.

Nutrition:

Calories: 131

Total Fat: 6g

Saturated Fat: 0g

Cholesterol: 0mg

Carbohydrates: 19g

Fiber: 3g

Protein: 3g

Phosphorus: 51mg

Potassium: 146mg

Sodium: 60mg

Blueberry Smoothie Bowl

Preparation Time: 5 minutes

Cooking Time: 0 minute

Servings: 1

Ingredients:

- ½ cup of frozen blueberries
- ½ cup of vanilla-flavored almond milk
- 1 tbsp. of agave syrup
- 1 tsp. of chia seeds

Directions:

1. Put all the ingredients in the blender except chia seeds, and blend until smooth. You should end up with a thick smoothie paste.
2. Transfer into a cereal bowl and top with chia seeds on top.

Nutrition:

Calories: 278.5

Carbohydrate: 38.72g

Protein: 1.3g

Sodium: 76.33mg

Potassium: 229.1mg

Phosphorus: 59.2mg

Dietary Fiber: 7.4g

Fat: 6g

Cucumber Green Smoothie

Preparation Time: 5 minutes

Cooking Time: 0 minute

Servings: 2

Ingredients:

- ½ cucumber, peeled and roughly chopped
- ½ green apple, roughly chopped
- 1 cup of Homemade Rice Milk or unsweetened store-bought rice milk
- 3 ice cubes

Directions:

1. In a blender, combine the cucumber, apple, milk, and ice.
2. Process until smooth, and serve.

Substitution tip: A tart green apple is lovely in this smoothie, as it creates a subtle sweetness. However, if you prefer, other apples, such as Fuji, Red Delicious, or McIntosh, can be used. If you are using a thick-skinned apple, peel it first for a nicer texture in the finished smoothie.

Nutrition:

Calories: 75

Total Fat: 2g

Saturated Fat: 0g

Cholesterol: 0mg

Carbohydrates: 14g

Fiber: 2g

Protein: 1g

Phosphorus: 34mg

Potassium: 313mg

Sodium: 81mg

Watermelon Kiwi Smoothie

Preparation Time: 5 minutes

Cooking Time: 0 minute

Servings: 2

Ingredients:

- 2 cups of watermelon chunks
- 1 kiwifruit, peeled
- 1 cup of ice

Directions:

1. In a blender, combine the watermelon, kiwi, and ice.
2. Process until smooth.

Nutrition tip: While watermelon tastes particularly sweet, it has only half the sugar of an apple. Because sugar is the main taste-producing element, it stands out the most. The other primary ingredient in watermelon is water.

Nutrition:

Calories: 67

Total Fat: 0g

Saturated Fat: 0g

Cholesterol: 0mg

Carbohydrates: 17g

Fiber: 2g

Protein: 1g

Phosphorus: 28mg

Potassium: 278mg

Sodium: 3mg

Mint Lassi

Preparation Time: 5 minutes

Cooking Time: 0 minute

Servings: 2

Ingredients:

- 1 teaspoon of cumin seeds
- ½ cup of mint leaves
- 1 cup of plain, unsweetened yogurt
- ½ cup of water

Directions:

1. In a skillet, toast cumin seeds until fragrant, 1 to 2 minutes in medium heat.
2. Transfer the seeds to a blender, along with the mint, yogurt, and water, and process until smooth.

Substitution tip: If you prefer the flavor of cilantro over mint, try it here instead. Another great substitute is to use ½ cup of strawberries along with ¼ teaspoon of ground cardamom instead of the mint.

Nutrition:

Calories: 114

Total Fat: 6g

Saturated Fat: 3g

Cholesterol: 15mg

Carbohydrates: 5g

Fiber: 0g

Protein: 10g

Phosphorus: 158mg

Potassium: 179mg

Sodium: 43mg

Fennel Digestive Cooler

Preparation Time: 5 minutes

Cooking Time: 15 minutes

Servings: 2

Ingredients:

- 2 cups Homemade Rice Milk or unsweetened store-bought rice milk
- ¼ cup fennel seeds, ground
- ¼ teaspoon ground cloves
- 1 tablespoon honey

Directions:

1. In a blender, combine the milk, fennel seeds, cloves, and honey.
2. Process until smooth, and let rest for 30 minutes.
3. Pour over a wire mesh strainer lined with cheesecloth or over a coffee filter set over a glass or jar.
4. Serve.

Nutrition tip: Fennel is a warming herb that is supportive of treating indigestion, gas, and hypertension. High in quercetin, an antioxidant flavonoid, fennel fights inflammation and inhibits the development of cancer, among other benefits.

Nutrition:

Calories: 163

Total Fat: 2g

Saturated Fat: 0g

Cholesterol: 0mg

Carbohydrates: 30g

Fiber: 5g

Protein: 3g

Phosphorus: 57mg

Potassium: 205mg

Sodium: 141mg

Cinnamon Horchata

Preparation Time: 5 minutes
Cooking Time: 0 minute
Servings: 5
Ingredients:
- 1 cup of long-grain white rice
- 4 cups of water
- 1 cinnamon stick, broken into pieces
- 1 cup of Homemade Rice Milk or unsweetened store-bought rice milk
- 1 teaspoon of vanilla extract
- 1 teaspoon of ground cinnamon
- 1/3cup of granulated sugar

Directions:
1. Using a blender, mix the rice, water, and cinnamon-stick pieces. For about 1 minute, blend until the rice begins to break up. Let stand at room temperature for at least 3 hours or overnight.
2. Place a wire mesh strainer over a pitcher, and pour the liquid into it. Discard the rice.
3. Add the milk, vanilla, ground cinnamon, and sugar. Stir to combine.
4. Serve over ice.

Variation tip: For an even richer flavor, add 1 tablespoon of unsweetened cocoa powder to the horchata with the ground cinnamon in Step 3.

Nutrition:
Calories: 123
Total Fat: 2g
Saturated Fat: 0g
Cholesterol: 0mg
Carbohydrates: 26g
Fiber: 0g
Protein: 1g
Phosphorus: 34mg
Potassium: 78mg
Sodium: 32mg

Vanilla Chia Smoothie

Preparation Time: 5 minutes
Cooking Time: 5 minutes
Servings: 2
Ingredients:

- 1 cup of Homemade Rice Milk or unsweetened store-bought rice milk
- 2 black tea bags
- 1 teaspoon of vanilla extract
- 1 cup of ice
- 1 teaspoon of honey
- 2 tablespoons of chia seeds
- ½ teaspoon of ground cinnamon
- ½ teaspoon of ground ginger
- ¼ teaspoon of ground cardamom
- ¼ teaspoon of ground cloves

Directions:

1. In a small pan, heat the rice milk to just steaming. Steep the tea bags for 5 minutes, then discard.

2. In a blender, combine the rice milk, vanilla, ice, honey, chia seeds, cinnamon, ginger, cardamom, and cloves. Process until smooth, and serve.

3. Substitution tip: To make this ahead, complete Step 1 and refrigerate the milk tea in an airtight container. When ready to make the smoothie, proceed as directed, reducing the ice to ½ cup and adding ¼ cup of water.

Nutrition:
Calories: 143
Total Fat: 5g
Saturated Fat: 1g
Cholesterol: 0mg
Carbohydrates: 19g
Fiber: 6g
Protein: 3g
Phosphorus: 3mg
Potassium: 93mg
Sodium: 73mg

Berry Mint Water

Preparation Time: 5 minutes

Cooking Time: 0 minute

Servings: 8

Ingredients:

- 8 cups of water
- ½ cup of strawberries
- ½ cup of blackberries
- 3 mint sprigs

Directions:

1. In a large pitcher, mix the water, strawberries, blackberries, and mint.
2. Cover and chill for at least 1 hour before drinking.
3. Store in the refrigerator for up to two days.

Substitution tip: Substitute any of your favorite fruits in this recipe to create your own flavored water. You can also try out different herbs to add bold and complementary flavors. Some additional herbs that taste nice paired with fruit include cilantro, basil, rosemary, and thyme. Ginger root is another favorite water flavor enhancer that stimulates digestion and cleanses the kidneys.

Nutrition:

Calories: 7

Total Fat: 0g

Saturated Fat: 0g

Cholesterol: 0mg

Carbohydrates: 2g

Fiber: 1g

Protein: 0g

Phosphorus: 4mg

Potassium: 28mg

Sodium: 0mg

Homemade Rice Milk

Preparation Time: 5 minutes

Cooking Time: 0 minute

Servings: 4

Ingredients:

- 1 cup of long-grain white rice
- 4 cups of water
- ½ teaspoon of vanilla extract (optional)

Directions:

1. In a dry skillet, set at medium heat, toast the rice until lightly browned, about 5 minutes.

2. Transfer the rice to a jar or bowl, and add the water. Cover, refrigerate and soak overnight.

3. In a blender, add the rice and water, along with the vanilla (if using), and process until smooth.

4. Place a fine-mesh strainer over a glass jar or bowl, and pour the milk into it. Serve immediately, or cover, refrigerate and serve within three days. Shake before using it.

Substitution tip: Rice milk can be substituted in most recipes calling for whole milk or another nut milk as a low-fat, low-phosphorus, and low-potassium alternative. Use an equal amount of rice milk in place of other milk products, and proceed as directed in the recipe.

Nutrition:

Calories: 112

Total Fat: 0g

Saturated Fat: 0g

Cholesterol: 0mg

Carbohydrates: 24g

Fiber: 0g

Protein: 0g

Phosphorus: 0mg

Potassium: 55mg

Sodium: 80mg

Ginger & Lemon Green Iced-Tea

Preparation Time: 5 minutes

Cooking Time: 0 minute

Servings: 2

Ingredients:

- 2 cups of concentrated green or matcha tea, served hot
- 1 lemon, cut into wedges
- 1/4 cup of crystallized ginger, chopped into fine pieces

Directions:

1. Get a glass container and mix the tea with the ginger and then cover and chill for 3 hours.
2. Strain and pour into serving glasses on top of ice if you wish.
3. Garnish with a wedge of lemon to serve.

Nutrition:

Calories: 20

Fat: 0g

Carbohydrates: 5g

Phosphorus: 9mg

Potassium: 106mg

Sodium: 4mg

Protein: 1g

Lemon Smoothie

Preparation Time: 5 minutes

Cooking Time: 0 minute

Servings: 2

Ingredients:

- 2 tbsp. of lemon juice
- 2 tbsp. of brown sugar or stevia
- 4 pasteurized liquid egg whites

Directions:

1. In a blender, combine all the ingredients. Process until smooth.
2. Garnish with a slice of lemon.

Nutrition:

Calories: 4

Fat: 0g

Carbohydrates: 5g

Phosphorus: 10mg

Potassium: 112mg

Sodium: 110mg

Protein: 8g

Tropical Juice

Preparation Time: 5 minutes

Cooking Time: 0 minute

Servings: 2

Ingredients:

- 2 cups of pineapple, chunks.
- 1/2 cup of low-fat coconut milk
- 1 cup of water

Directions:

1. In a blender, combine all the ingredients. Process until smooth.

2. Serve immediately.

Tip: Check with your doctor or dietitian as to whether you can still have coconut milk. Alternatively, use non-dairy milk, such as almond.

Nutrition:

Calories: 55

Fat: 9g

Carbohydrates: 6g

Phosphorus: 11mg

Potassium: 129mg

Sodium: 111mg

Protein: 7g

Mixed Fruit Anti-Inflammatory Smoothie

Preparation Time: 5 minutes

Cooking Time: 0 minute

Servings: 4

Ingredients:

- 1 cup of red or white grapes
- 1 cup of sliced frozen or fresh peaches
- 1 cup of chopped cabbage
- 1/2 cup of ice cubes
- 1/2 cup of water
- 1 sprig of fresh mint

Directions:

1. In a blender, combine all the ingredients. Process until smooth.
2. Serve immediately in tall glasses.
3. Tear mint with fingers and serve with smoothies (optional).

Nutrition:

Calories: 48

Fat: 0g

Carbohydrates: 12g

Phosphorus: 17mg

Potassium: 203mg

Sodium: 6mg

Protein: 1g

Winter Berry Iced Milkshake

Preparation Time: 5 minutes

Cooking Time: 0 minute

Servings: 4

Ingredients:

- 1 cup of rice milk, unenriched
- 1/2 cup of organic blueberries (or washed if non-organic)
- 1/2 cup of blackberries
- Ice cubes to the desired concentration

Direction:

1. Add ingredients together in a blender, blending until smooth, and then serve in tall glasses.

Nutrition:

Calories: 45

Fat: 1g

Carbohydrates: 7g

Phosphorus: 33mg

Potassium: 118mg

Sodium: 29mg

Protein: 2g

Aloha Cocktail

Preparation Time: 10 minutes

Cooking Time: 0 minute

Servings: 2

Ingredients:

- 1 cup of fresh pineapple cubes
- 1 lime cut in half and juiced
- ½ cup of ginger ale
- Ice cubes

Directions:

2. Place pineapple, lime juice, and ginger ale in the blender.
3. Blend until smooth.
4. Pour into a glass filled with ice.

Nutrition:

Calories: 63.5

Protein: 0.4g

Sodium: 5.4mg

Phosphorus: 0.8mg

Potassium: 110.4mg

Almonds & Blueberries Smoothie

Preparation time: 5 minutes

Cooking time: 3 minutes

Servings: 2

Ingredients:

- 1/4 cup ground almonds, unsalted
- 1 cup fresh blueberries
- Fresh juice of a 1 lemon
- 1 cup fresh kale leaf
- 1/2 cup coconut water
- 1 cup water
- 2 tablespoon plain yogurt (optional)

Directions:

1. Dump all ingredients in your high-speed blender, and blend until your smoothie is smooth.

2. Pour the mixture in a chilled glass.

3. Serve and enjoy!

Nutrition:

Calories: 110,

Carbohydrates: 8g,

Proteins: 2g,

Fat: 7g,

Fiber: 2g,

Calcium 19mg,

Phosphorous 16mg,

Potassium 27mg

Sodium: 101 m

Almonds and Zucchini Smoothie

Preparation time: 5 minutes

Cooking time: 3 minutes

Servings: 2

Ingredients:

- 1 cup zucchini, cooked and mashed - unsalted
- 1 1/2 cups almond milk
- 1 tablespoon almond butter (plain, unsalted)
- 1 teaspoon pure almond extract
- 2 tablespoon ground almonds or macadamia almonds
- 1/2 cup water
- 1 cup ice cubes crushed (optional, for serving)

Directions:

1. Dump all ingredients from the list above in your fast-speed blender; blend for 45 - 60 seconds or to taste.

2. Serve with crushed ice.

Nutrition:

Calories: 322,

Carbohydrates: 6g,

Proteins: 6g,

Fat: 30g,

Fiber: 3.5g

Calcium 9mg,

Phosphorous 26mg,

Potassium 27mg

Sodium: 121 mg

Blueberries and Coconut Smoothie

Preparation time: 5 minutes

Cooking time: 3 minutes

Servings: 5

Ingredients:

- 1 cup of frozen blueberries, unsweetened
- 1 cup stevia or erythritol sweetener
- 2 cups coconut milk (canned)
- 2 tablespoon shredded coconut (unsweetened)
- 3/4 cup water

Directions:

1. Place all ingredients from the list in food-processor or in your strong blender.
2. Blend for 45 - 60 seconds or to taste.
3. Ready for drink! Serve!

Nutrition:

Calories: 190,

Carbohydrates: 8g,

Proteins: 3g,

Fat: 18g,

Fiber: 2g,

Calcium 79mg,

Phosphorous 216mg,

Potassium 207mg

Sodium: 121 mg

Creamy Dandelion Greens and Celery Smoothie

Preparation time: 10 minutes

Cooking time: 3 minutes

Servings: 2

Ingredients:

- 1 handful of raw dandelion greens
- 2 celery sticks
- 2 tablespoon chia seeds
- 1 small piece of ginger, minced
- 1/2 cup almond milk
- 1/2 cup of water
- 1/2 cup plain yogurt

Directions:

1. Rinse and clean dandelion leaves from any dirt; add in a high-speed blender.

2. Clean the ginger; keep only inner part and cut in small slices; add in a blender.

3. Blend all remaining ingredients until smooth.

4. Serve and enjoy!

Nutrition:

Calories: 58,

Carbohydrates: 5g,

Proteins: 3g,

Fat: 6g,

Fiber: 3g

Calcium 29mg,

Phosphorous 76mg,

Potassium 27mg

Sodium: 121 mg

CPSIA information can be obtained
at www.ICGtesting.com
Printed in the USA
BVHW061059030521
606339BV00010B/1597